T0315293

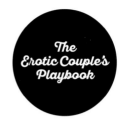

The Erotic Couple's Playbook

Awesome Oral

QUIVER

Contents

Part 1
Pussy Play

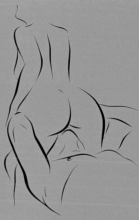

Part 2
How to Cock Please

First, a Little Anatomy Lesson

1. **Vulva**: All the parts on the outside of a woman's genitals, including the lips, clitoris, mons, vaginal opening, and urethral opening. Sometimes when people say "vagina" they mean "vulva."

2. **Labia majora**: The large fleshy lips on either side of the inner labia which may be covered in pubic hair.

3. **Labia minora**: Hairless lips that range in color from light pink to a dark brownish black and in size from small to prominent. They're sensitive and swell when aroused.

4. **Mons or Venus mound**: The soft area of fatty tissue above the pubic bone which may be covered in hair.

5. **Clitoris**: Most people think of the clitoris as the tip but it's actually an extensive structure of erectile tissue, both internal and external, including a head, hood, shaft, bulbs, and legs. It swells when aroused and is designed solely for pleasure.

6. **Clitoral head**: This highly sensitive tip is located at the top of the vulva where the inner lips meet. Most people need some sort of clitoral stimulation—direct or indirect, depending on owner—to reach orgasm.

7. **Clitoral hood**: A bit of foreskin that covers and protects the clitoral head. It may retract when the clitoral head swells.

8. **Clitoral shaft**: Attached to the clitoral head, when erect it wraps around the vagina on the inside of the body.

9. **Clitoral legs**: Two long internal legs that form a V-shape around the vaginal walls and urethra.

10. **Clitoral bulbs**: Located internally beneath the outer labia, these internal bulbs swell with arousal and cause the rhythmic contractions during orgasms.

11. **Vagina**: This tubelike canal is composed of mucous membranes and enclosed by elastic tissue and muscles. Vaginas can be penetrated with toys, a penis, or fingers. Some people like rhythmic pressure against the top wall of the vagina, an area some people call the G-spot but is now considered part of the internal clitoris.

12. **Urethral opening**: The tiny hole below the clitoris where urine and ejaculate come out.

13. **Anus**: A.K.A., the butt hole. As it is filled with sensitive nerve endings, many people like anal stimulation with a finger, the mouth, toys, or penetration. (Note: The anus and rectum are not self-lubricating, so with any anal play, make sure to use a lot of lube and go slowly.)

14. **Perineum**: The smooth area of skin, also called the taint, between the lower vulva and the anus. Some people like a tongue, a vibrator, or a finger pressed against it.

The Vulva and
Surrounding Areas

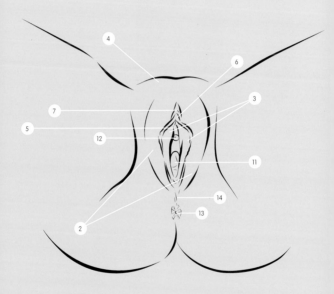

Yer a Peach

01

Because they are so very yummy

Show your partner exactly how sweet you think they taste by burying your face between their legs and using your mouth on them like you'd eat a peach. Cover your teeth with your lips, then grab your partner's butt cheeks and pull them close to your mouth. Wrap your lips around the outer edges of their vulva. Be messy as you suck, as though you're relishing the best, juiciest peach. Because you are. Go ahead and let them know that.

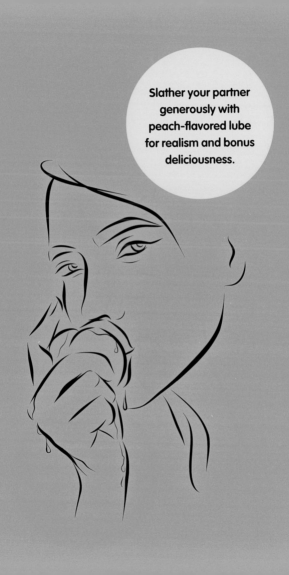

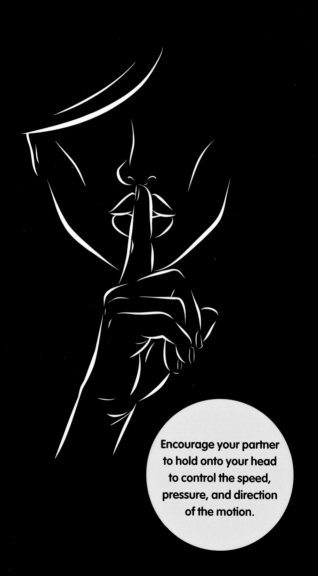

Yes and No

02

Use your head

Use the motion of your head to complement the stimulation of your mouth and tongue by placing your mouth over your partner's clit. Shake your head back and forth in a "no" motion, using a bit of suction. Intersperse with an up and down "yes" motion using your tongue to lick up the length of clit or entire vulva. As they get closer to orgasm, switch to just one method to put them over the edge.

Yasss Queen(ing)

03

This seat open?

Lie on your back with your partner straddling your face. They slide their vulva over your mouth, using your lips and face as they please. Press your tongue to their clit, purse your lips out firmly, shake your head slowly back and forth, or just lie back and take it. Note: Even though this move is called "face sitting," have your partner go with more of a hover than a full sit, so it feels less suffocating.

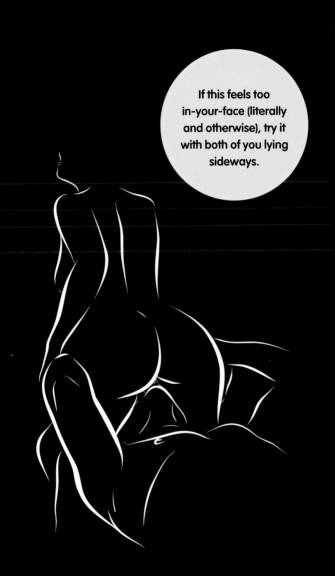

The Peace Out

04

Keep the peace in your bedroom

Adding your fingers to oral gives you lots more options for loving up your partner. In The Peace Out, place two well-lubed fingers on each side of your partner's clit. You can press your fingers together to make the clit head jut out a little or slide them loosely up and down each side. Bring your mouth into it with long licks up their vulva or focus your pointed tongue on and around the head of their clit.

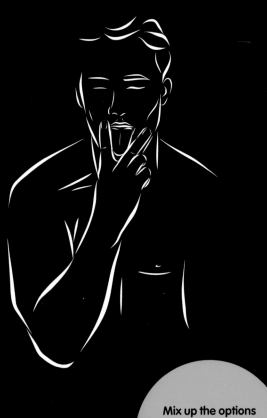

Mix up the options for your mouth and fingers to create bonus new moves.

Make sure your partner knows that you f-ing *love* what you're doing, and you're golden.

The Cat Lady

05

Me-ow

Lap up your partner's pussy like a cat licking up a rich bowl of cream. Lie your partner on their back and kneel, hooking their legs over your shoulders. Bend down about an inch from their pussy and linger for a moment, letting them feel your warm breath. Start with long licks up their vulva, gradually working more rhythmically using long firm tongue strokes.

A Side of Oral

06

The Kivin method is for foolproof orgasm, at least according to TikTok

Behold the wisdom of the Kivin method, a kind of sideways oral that magically makes everything better. To do it, come in from the side, kneeling by your partner's hips. Grasp their clit on both sides with a finger and thumb. Use your mouth to sweep from side to side, so you're going up and down the clit from an entirely different angle, covering lots of clitoral real estate. Tart it up with finger on their perineum.

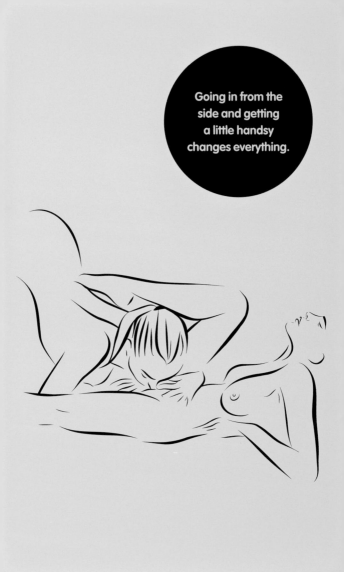

Going in from the side and getting a little handsy changes everything.

Hey, Squirt

07

How to (try) to wrangle the elusive phenomenon that is squirting

No promises—squirting (female ejaculation) doesn't happen for everyone, or even for most people. But to create squirting-conducive conditions, start by getting your partner well aroused. Suck on their clit and slide two fingers into their vagina. Stroke on the upper wall, alternating a come hither motion with side to side rubbing. A G-spot toy can be a huge help here too. There *may* be squirting. And there may not. All good either way.

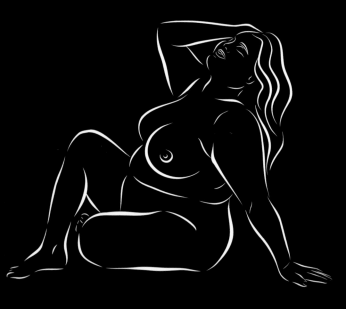

To encourage squirting, try pressing rhythmically with a flat hand on the area above the mons (the fleshy pubic bone area).

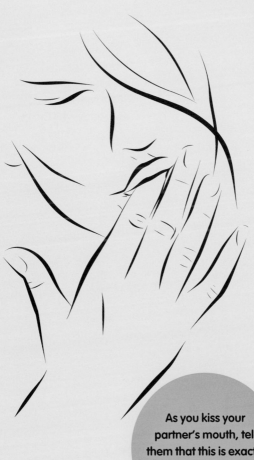

As you kiss your partner's mouth, tell them that this is exactly how you're doing to go down on them.

Kissy Face

08

It's like a French kiss for the pussy

Give their pussy the love it deserves with a full-on make-out session. Start with a languid kissing session, using your tongue to give a preview of what awaits them below. With your tongue leading the way, move on down to their vulva. Kiss all over their vulva—outer lips, inner lips, and clit. Use your tongue for long licks up your partner's inner lips, slide your tongue inside their vagina, and make back and forth sweeps over their clit.

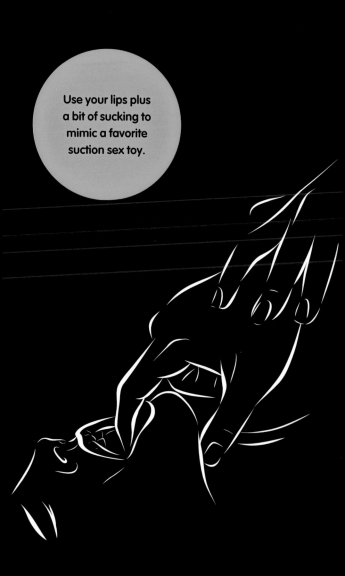

Use your lips plus a bit of sucking to mimic a favorite suction sex toy.

The Human Sex Toy

09

Are you better than your partner's favorite sex toy? Damn right.

Clit suction vibrators are hugely popular for a reason—they give a highly focused but gentle stimulation that doesn't usually occur in the wild. Use this wisdom to your advantage. Become your partner's personal clit suction toy by copying the exact motion. Purse your lips around then suck very gently around—not on—the tip of the clit. Suck softly and rhythmically, adjusting speed according to your partner's moans. It's like a wee little blow job, but for clits.

Giving Head

10

Can you take instruction?

Let your partner decide what kind of stimulation they want by giving them complete control. For this, your partner sits at the edge of a bed or chair. Kneel between their legs with your face pressed to their vulva. Your partner holds your head between their legs, moving it as they please. They can just control the pressure, speed, and movement with their hands or tweak it with verbal instructions like "wiggle your tongue, pleeeease" or "OMG, more sucking."

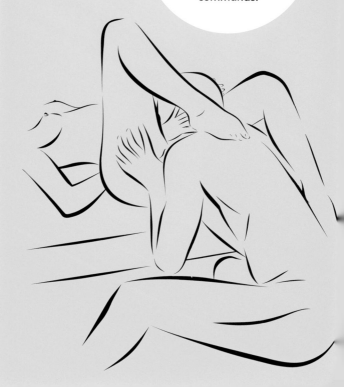

For a more dominant/submissive vibe, kneel before your partner while they stand. All the better to obey their commands.

The Nose Job

11

Put your nose to excellent use

During oral sex, the nose is right there, next to the action, but is usually consigned to the oral sex bench. Get it into the game by playing to its strengths. It's firm, it juts out in a fetching manner, and, like we said, it's already right there. Slide your tongue around the entrance to the vagina and inside. Use your nose to make circles around the clit, rub side to side, or go up one side and down the other.

Put a dollop of lube on the tip of your nose to make it glide more smoothly.

Press two thumbs
on either side of their
clit to add a firm
contrast to the light
flickering motion
of your tongue.

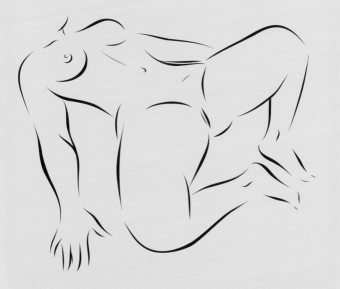

The Butterfly

12

Spread their "wings," like you're in a GD 1970s hippie song

Start the butterfly by having your partner butterfly their legs in a lying down version of the butterfly stretch in gym class—feet together, knees bent and splayed to the sides. Spread open the lips to their vulva and hold them open. Flick your tongue back and forth, lightly and rapidly, teasing their clit. As they get closer to orgasm, you can press more firmly with your tongue or stick with what's already working.

Beg for It

13

Anticipation makes everything *so* much better

Make your partner crave your mouth before you give it to them. Kiss them all over their body, but before you move to a new part, make them ask for it, i.e., "Do you want me to suck on your earlobes?" "Kiss your neck?" "Lick your nipples?" Lick and nibble your way up their thighs then tease them by brushing your mouth around their pussy, but not on. Keep it up until they can't think of anything but your mouth. On them. Now.

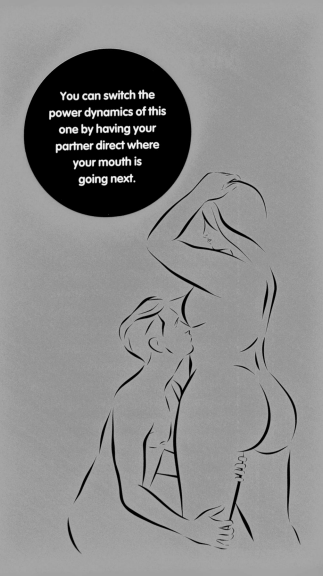

Mirror, Mirror

14

Y'all look GOOD

Indulge your voyeurism and exhibitionist tendencies at the same time by going down on your partner in front of a mirror. Adjust according to fetish: If they like to watch and you don't, they face the mirror and you don't. If you're both hardcore exhibitionists, do a full-on performance for yourselves. If anyone has any body image stuff going on (it happens, that societal crap is insidious!), set up some candles to give yourselves an instant gorgeousness upgrade.

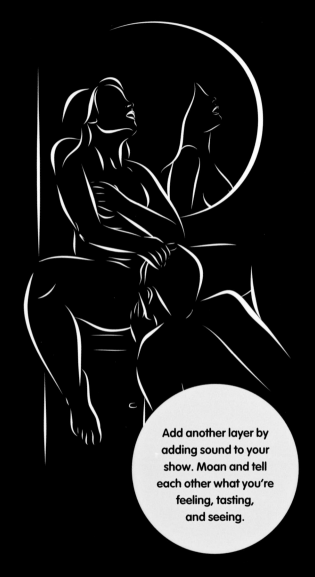

Add another layer by adding sound to your show. Moan and tell each other what you're feeling, tasting, and seeing.

If your partner is game, try using a cooling or warming lube for extra sensations.

Cup a Lube

15

How to tame a pussy

Fill your hand with lube and have your partner go on all fours with you kneeling behind. Cup your lube-filled hand under their vulva and rub, pressing your palm over their vulva and letting your fingers slide over and alongside their clit. You can also hold your hand steady while they take control by rocking their hips. If they want more pressure, have them lie face down with their hips on a pillow to hump your slippery hand.

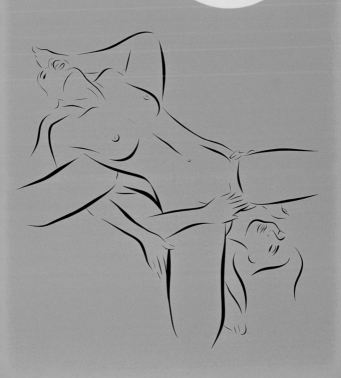

The New 69... the 68

16

It's like 69 minus the multitasking

68 sounds way more complicated than it actually is, so pay attention: Lie on your back with your knees bent. Your partner lies onto top of you, facing up, with their back resting on your bent legs so that their crotch is conveniently by your mouth. Reach around their hips to hold onto them. Without the multitasking of 69, you'll be better able to focus on what you're doing. And they can return the favor later.

Tantric Oral

17

Slow it waaaay down

A big part of tantric sex is being completely in the moment with your partner, savoring every breath and movement. The best way to get to that kind of mindfulness is to slow way down. Try it with some extremely slo-mo oral. Go very slowly, to the degree that it seems like you might be going *too* slowly. Meaning, take 20 seconds to lick up the length of your partner's vulva. You'll both be uber-focused on your every little move.

Try a lube with CBD in it. The CBD helps increase blood flow and makes everything feel like just… more.

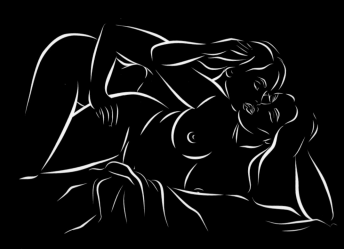

G-spot toys don't require thrusting. Just press, tap, or rub it gently against the upper wall of the vagina.

The Purring Kitty

18

Toy + your mouth = OMG

Sucking on your partner's clit is all kinds of good, but adding a toy to the mix will put them over the top. Get their vulva and clit warmed up with your finest oral moves. Lick their vulva, make circles around their clit, and suck gently. Find good rhythm or type of stimulation—this will be your finishing move. Lube up a G-spot toy, slide it inside their vagina, and fire it up. Let it hum away while you work on their clit.

Shake It Off

19

A bit of suction makes a huge difference

Put your mouth around your partner's clit and suck in to create suction. Since your lips are around and not on the clitoral head, you can use a lot of suction (obvs. see how your partner is feeling about it.) While keeping the suction going, shake your head back and forth—gently or vigorously, up to you. The combination of the two sensations at once is intense though, so only bust out this move when it's orgasm time.

Create a triple sensation by adding flicks of your tongue.

In Your Face

20

It's like Queening lite

Sit up in bed, leaning back on a comfortable stack of pillows, with your legs out in front of you. And that's kinda it. You can hold onto their ass, but otherwise your work here is pretty much done. Your partner straddles you, kneeling in front of your face. They press their vulva onto your open mouth and basically hump your face. It's like Queening, but with less intense pussy engulfment.

If you want to
be more than
a pretty face
to f*ck, point
your tongue out
stiffly to give
your partner
a penetrative
option.

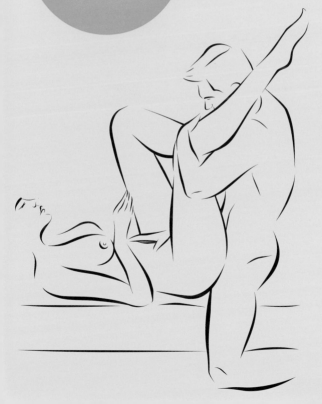

For a variation, instead of having your partner say what they want, have them guide you with their hands.

As You Wish

21

Your partner tells you what to do. You do it.

Let your partner run the show. Have them lie back, open their legs, then tell you what they want you to do with your mouth. The more specific they are, the better it will be for the both of you. "Suck very gently on the tip of my clit" is better than "Suck me." Not only will you be giving them exactly the kind of stimulation they want, as they want it, but you are collecting valuable intel for what their particular pussy likes.

Ask them to show you how they touch themselves then mimic that motion with your mouth.

Jilling Off

22

Fun(ish) fact: The vulva-centric term for jacking off is jilling off

Everyone's different and all that, but a super common way that people with vulvas touch themselves is by using a few fingers to rub their clit back and forth. You can mimic that motion by pressing your tongue flat over their clit. Go ahead and press decently hard—unless you get feedback otherwise, your flat tongue won't be too much. Shake your head to the left and right, gliding your tongue over their clit. Add a little tongue wiggle for extra finesse.

The Pussy Puppet

23

Give yourself a hand

Your mouth can do all kinds of glorious things to a pussy, but it can't do everything, at least not all at once. So get your hand involved. Start by giving the clit some love with licks, sucks, and tongue flicks. See what's working for you and settle in with that. Then slide a well-lubed finger in your partner's butt and a lubey thumb in their vagina. (Or vice versa, assess your own hand ergonomics.) Slide, thrust, and wiggle your fingers inside them.

You can use either a finger or thumb in the butt, but decide whichever digit is "butt only" to avoid transferring bacteria to the vagina.

Double Pleasure

24

Penetration and your mouth FTW

Mixing up types of stimulation is a great way to enhance both. This does that, but also has an animalistic vibe, which makes it feel a little more raw and dirty. Have your partner on all fours. Get on your knees behind them and switch between sucking their vulva and penetrating them with penis or dildo. Get them close to orgasm, but not *quite* there, then, when they can't take it, let them choose which way you're gonna make them come.

If you want to add a little consensual BDSM, add a few swats on the butt in there.

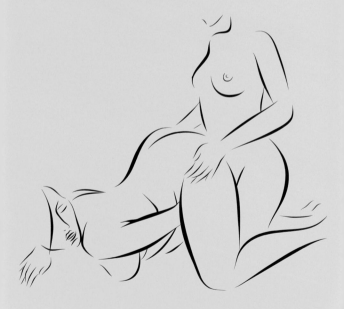

Butty Love

25

Analingus plus rabbit vibe equals big-ass orgasm

Analingus, a.k.a. a rim job or rimming, is oral sex for the butt hole. If y'all are into analingus, you know that it's plenty fun but not necessarily an orgasmic kind of fun. Rectify that by adding an orgasm-inducing rabbit vibrator. Your partner holds the rabbit vibe while it works its magic against their clit and inside their vagina. You're on butt duty. Make small circles around their butthole with your tongue, interspersed with licks, kisses, and gentle sucking.

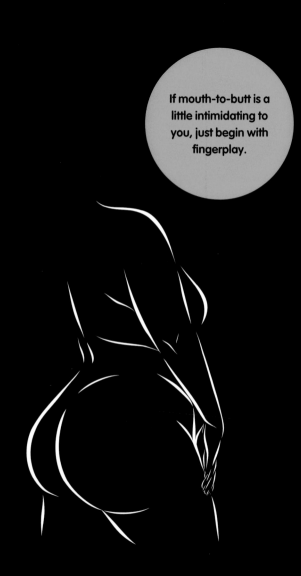

If your partner's signed off on it beforehand, chill the dildo ahead of time for extra feelz.

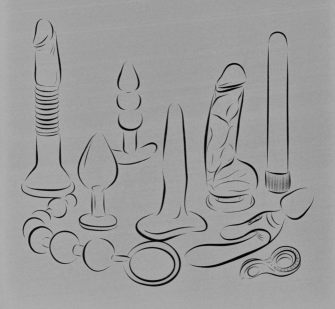

Oh. My. God.

26

Press a dildo against the area that is not called the G-spot

Yes, the "G-spot" is not a separate thing and is actually just part of the extensive clitoral internal structure and all that. And yet. For a lot of people, having something pressed against it when they're well turned on can help bring about truly epic orgasms. See for yourself. As your mouth brings your partner closer to orgasm, slide a curved glass or metal dildo inside their vagina. Press and slide it against the upper wall of their vagina, using a firm pressure.

Emerge from between their legs a few times to kiss them and give them a taste of themselves.

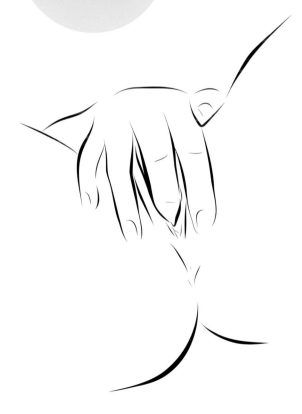

The Mix Master

27

You're the lube bartender

Loving the taste of your partner is part of really great sex. But if you want to mix it up once in a while, use flavored lubes. Be a baller and mix flavored lubes to create new tastes between their legs. Try apple + caramel = caramel apple! Salted caramel + mocha java = caramel macchiato! The flavor play options are endless.

Wait for It

28

It's frustrating, but in a good way

Edging is bringing a partner *just* to the brink of orgasm, then stopping so that when you finally do take them over the edge, the results are explosive. To do it, ply your partner's clit and vulva with your mouth and tongue. Settle upon a rhythm that gets them very close to an orgasm, then stop for a moment to let their desire ebb slightly. Repeat, repeat, repeat until your partner can't think of anything besides how much they need to come.

Get familiar with the signs that your partner is extremely close to orgasm, i.e., heavy breathing, straining toward your mouth, incoherent begging.

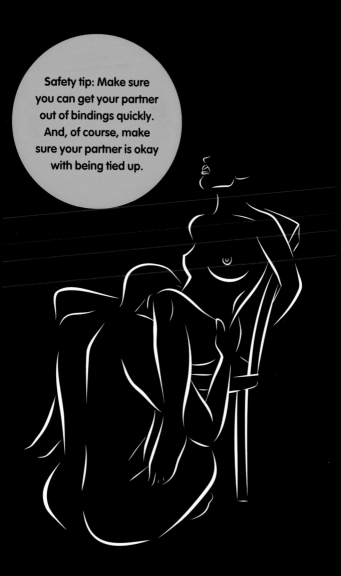

Safety tip: Make sure you can get your partner out of bindings quickly. And, of course, make sure your partner is okay with being tied up.

Sit Down. Now.

29

Obeying and being obeyed can be super hot

Sit your partner down with their wrists bound behind them. If you don't have handcuffs, DIY it using a necktie, scarf, or an old t-shirt. Hold your partner's legs open. If you're feeling dramatic, behold their pussy for a long moment, and tell them exactly what you're going to do to it and how much you're going to love it. Keep their legs pried open and use your thumbs to massage open their lips while sucking on their clit.

The Figure Eight

30

Numbers > Letters

The "spelling the alphabet with your tongue" technique *seems* like it would work because it covers a lot of clitoral real estate, and if you want to do that as a warm-up move, go to town. But actual orgasms come from consistent and rhythmic stimulation. Trace your partner's clit with your tongue in a figure-8 motion. Travel around the bottom of the clitoral shaft and over the top, crossing at their clitoral head. Hold their thighs open with your hands and massage them while you're figure 8-ing.

Switch this up by turning it on its side and drawing an infinity symbol with your tongue.

First, a Little Anatomy Lesson

1. **Head**: Also known as the tip or the glans, this is the bulbous part at the end of the shaft and is the most sensitive part of the penis. It also contains the opening to the urethra, the small hole where pre-ejaculate (pre-cum), semen, and urine come out.

2. **Shaft**: The shaft is the main part of the penis between the head and where it connects to the body. It looks like a tube and is made of spongey tissue that expands during erections.

3. **Corona**: This is the flared ridge surrounding the base of the head. It responds to touch and swells during arousal.

4. **Frenulum**: The little piece of connective tissue on the underside of the penis at the top of the shaft and base of the head. It's very sensitive to direct stimulation.

5. **Foreskin**: The protective layer of skin that covers the head of the penis. If a person has been circumcised, the foreskin has been removed and the head is more visible. If the person is uncircumcised, the head is partially covered with the foreskin. Uncircumcised people often have more sensitivity in their penis.

6. **Testicles**: Commonly known as balls, they're inside the scrotal sac and produce sperm cells. They're extremely sensitive to pain. They retract closer to the body via a muscle called the cremaster when a person is cold or nearing orgasm.

7. **Scrotum**: Also known as the ball sack, this is the soft skin sac that contain the testicles. Some people like gentle touches, tugs, and licks on the scrotum.

8. **Perineum**: A.K.A., the taint, this is the sensitive space between the anus and the base of the scrotum. Some people like a tongue, a vibrator, or a finger pressed against it.

9. **Prostate**: Also called the P-spot, the prostate is an internal walnut-shaped gland. It can be accessed by pressing against the upper wall of the rectum with hand or toy. Stimulating it can give some people a "p-gasm," which can feel deeper and produce more ejaculate.

10. **Anus**: A.K.A., the butt hole. It has lots of sensitive nerve endings, and many people like anal stimulation with a finger, the mouth, toys, or penetration. (Note: The anus and rectum are not self-lubricating, so with any anal play, make sure to use a lot of lube and go slowly.)

The Penis and Surrounding Areas

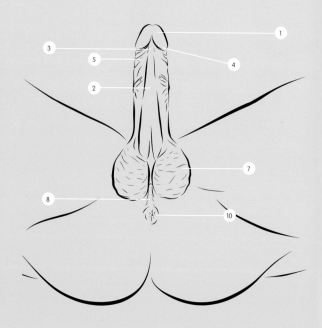

The Corkscrew

01

A BJ with a twist

This is insanely easy and gets a big reaction for little effort, a plus for any sex tip. Start with your lips around the head of your partner's cock. Travel down to the base, twisting your head from side to side. Suck up and down the shaft, twisting your head as you go and letting your tongue trail along. Slow down at the frenulum to give it a few extra loving flicks of your tongue.

Try adding a zig-zagging motion with your tongue as you travel up and down the shaft.

The 7 and 1

02

When you need a plan

If you set up a predictable rhythm, you and your partner can both relax into the experience and the sensations. Put your mouth around your partner's penis with your two hands circling the base. Use your hands and mouth to stroke up the shaft and head seven times. Then reverse the motion with a firm downstroke once. Repeat the sequence, seven up, one down.

As they get closer to orgasm, switch to a one up and one down stroke.

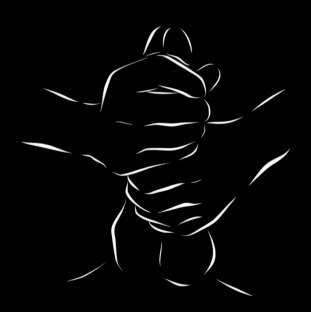

F Is for Frenulum

03

Make friends with the frenulum

Spend some quality time with the frenulum, the sensitive spot on the underside of the penis where the head and the shaft meet. To give it some focused attention, lube your hands up and wrap them around the base of your partner's cock. Lower your mouth on the head of their cock, then slide your tongue out against the underside of the head, sweeping it back and forth as you suck gently with your lips. Add a head twist if you're feeling it.

Be extra:
Alternate
between using
the top side of
your tongue
to stroke the
frenulum
wand then the
underside of
tongue on the
upper side of
the head.

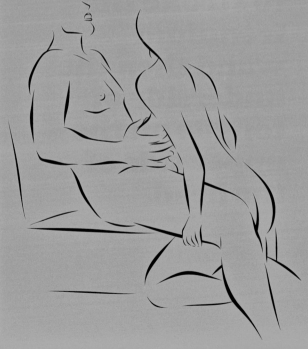

The Super Soaker

04

Incoming! Let your partner choose where they want to ejaculate

If your partner gets off on coming on a certain place (your chest, your lips, in your mouth, whatever), let them choose the area of honor. As they get closer, look them in the eye, aiming them toward said area of honor. Some people love if you say stuff like, "I want you to come on my (wherever)," some don't. Figure out who you have and act accordingly. (If you want the exact opposite of this and want any cum geysers contained, use your hand to cover their head as they're ejaculating.)

Either partner can be in control here—the owner of the penis with their thrusting, or you with your mouth and head motions.

The Side Car

05

A BJ that can be done on a fainting couch

Feeling lazy? Bust out the side car. Lie on a bed with your head turned to the side at the edge of the bed. Your partner stands beside the bed, leaning with their hands on the bed to adjust the dick-to-mouth height. Use your hand to direct their penis into your mouth, using the other hand to hold onto their butt to control their thrusts. The result? A fine BJ while you're lying down comfortably. Good for folks with movement restrictions, too.

Mr. Cocky

06

Put a ring on it

Cock rings work by trapping blood in the penis to create harder, longer-lasting erections, enhanced sensations, and more powerful orgasms. (It also makes penises look bigger which is just aesthetics, but isn't nothing.) Harness these powers for good by having your partner wear a cock ring during a blow job. Get a stretchy ring and wrap it around the base of the shaft or around the base and behind the balls. Perform your usual BJ magic and it'll all be just a little better.

If you don't have a cock ring on hand, DIY one by wrapping your hands around the base of the penis and behind the balls.

The Face F*ck

07

It's what it sounds like

If you want to muck about with power dynamics, kneel before your partner (this is inherently a subservient position) and let them thrust into your mouth. They're basically using your mouth to give themselves a blow job, so make sure that's cool with you and if, at any point, it becomes super uncool, stop. If you need a little buffer, circle your hand around their shaft so they can't go too deep.

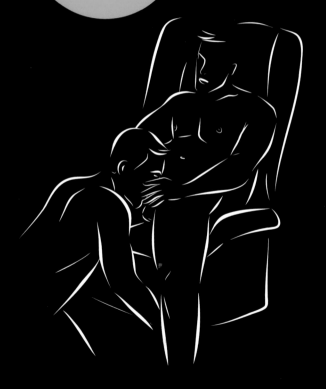

For an even more hard-core dynamic, lie on your back and let your partner have their way with your mouth.

Make the sleeve as warm and inviting as your mouth by filling it with a warming lube.

The Pop Up

08

Bring in a penis sleeve for backup

Penis sleeves, a.k.a. masturbators or strokers, are usually a solo kind of deal, but they are excellent as part of a well-balanced BJ. Fill a stroker with lube and slide it over your partner's penis. (It doesn't matter if they are hard or not. They will be.) Take advantage of the tight fit of the penis sleeve and use it to stroke their shaft. At the same time, suck on their head, synching the movement of your hand and mouth.

The Porn Star

09

Oh yeah, baby

Be your partner's in-home porn star by porning it up for them. Co-opt the hottest and/or cheesiest moves from mainstream porn. Look up into their eyes as you suck on their penis. Use a *lot* of spit. Press their cock into your cheek with your tongue so they can see the outline of themselves in your mouth. Take them deeply into your mouth and let yourself gag a bit. (This is all consensual and a bit of theater.)

Let your partner choose some BJ porn then reenact it move by move.

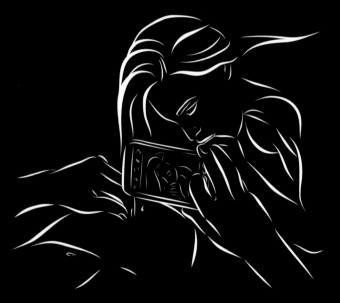

Opposite Day

10

Switch it up

Lube up your hands and circle the middle of your partner's shaft. Use one hand to stroke up, and the other one down. At the same time, use your mouth to focus on their head. Lick around the rim of the head, flick the frenulum with your tongue and/or suck and lick the head. As they get closer to orgasm, switch to just sucking the head and a strong and steady stroke with your hands.

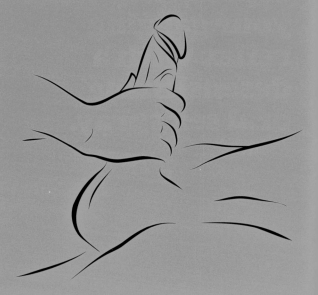

If you want
to go deep but
hate the gagging
aspect, help tame
your gagging
reflex with a
desensitizing
oral sex spray.

Deep Throating

11

Here's your deep throating 101

Deep throating is taking your partner's entire cock into your mouth then swallowing around their penis. This can make you gag. Totally normal, and if that's okay with you, lean into it. A lot of people like the gagging aspect of it because it makes contractions around the head of the penis that feel good, plus it's a little porny. If you're not into gagging, wrap your hand around the base of their penis to prevent them from going too deep.

Deep(ish) Throat

12

It's okay to fake it

If your gag reflex doesn't allow for a full-on deep throating, you have options. **1.** As you suck, turn your head, letting the head of their penis press against the inside of your cheek. It feels similar to them, but less gaggy for you. **2.** Use your hand as an extension of your mouth. Create a tight suction around your partner's shaft with your hands, pressing them next to your mouth for a seamless feel. Voila!

Warm some lube between your hands to enhance the illusion of a hot mouth.

Put your hands against your partner's hips so you can control the depth of penetration.

Deepest Throat

13

Plumb the depths

If deep throating isn't quite deep enough, you can go *even* deeper. Lie on a bed with your head leaning back over a pillow or the edge of the bed. They stand or kneel to enter your mouth. Take them as deeply as you into your mouth. If you can take them up to the base, that's great. If you can't, use your hand as a mouth extension. Alternate between sucking up and down their shaft and swallowing around them.

The Slip and Slide

14

It's a classic for a reason, okay to fake it

Regardless of what you've got going on up top, you can give a great titty fuck. The secret is to use your hands to supplement boobs/moobs. Start by lying back with your partner straddling you. Press your lubed up boobs/moobs around the side of their penis and wrap your hands around the rest of their shaft to encircle their penis with your bounty. Take the head of their penis in your mouth and let them thrust away.

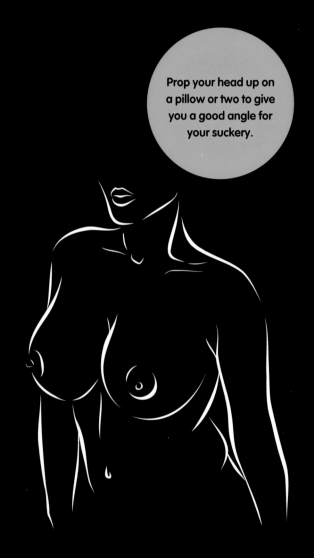

Yes, Master

15

You will do as they please

Your partner gives you instructions, you follow them. Let your partner control *exactly* how you use your mouth on them. Have them direct the whole experience, from how you first touch their body to how you make them come. Not only do you get to play with dominance and submission, which can be super hot, but you get a private oral sex lesson on how to please them. For an extra subservient vibe, get on your knees in front of them.

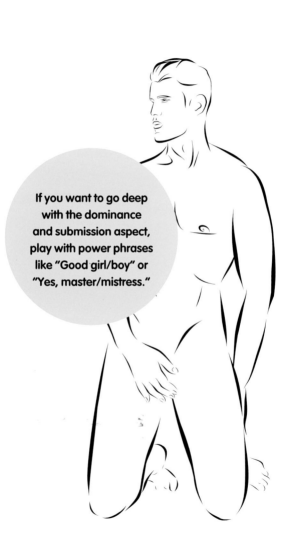

If you want to go deep with the dominance and submission aspect, play with power phrases like "Good girl/boy" or "Yes, master/mistress."

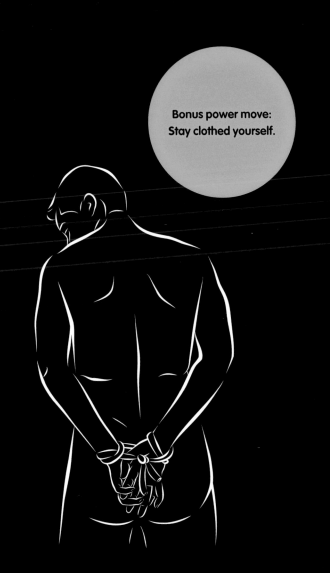

Lie Your Booty Down

16

You heard me

Sit your partner in a hard, straight-backed chair like a dining chair and restrain their wrists behind them with handcuffs or bindings. You can unzip their pants or have them be completely naked, depending on the level of vulnerability they're comfortable with, provided they're cool with being restrained in the first place. Use your mouth and hands to bring them to the brink of orgasm then stop, leaving them frustrated (in a good way) that they can't touch you or themselves. Repeat as needed, until the begging starts.

Kneel at their side for aesthetics (the view of your fine self) and to give extra stim to the frenulum.

So Cheeky

17

Put your cheeks to work for you

Get your cheeks involved in a blow job to give your partner completely new sensations. Press your tongue flat against the bottom of your mouth to cover your bottom teeth and lower your lips over their head. Suck your cheeks in so they're pressing against your partner's cock. Move your mouth up and down their shaft and head, maintaining the suction. If (when) your cheeks get tired, press your hands against your cheeks to keep the tight feel.

The Suck Up

18

Suck up, not down

To focus your partner's attention on your every move, switch up the sensations. Grasp the base of their penis firmly with your thumb and fingers. Put your mouth as far down as it will go to the base of their penis, then suck your way up the shaft and head. Slide back down, but just use your lips, no suction. The downstroke won't feel *quite* as good as the upstroke, so when that upstroke hits, it's extra good.

As they get closer
to orgasm, be
nice and switch
to suction for
both directions.

Head of the Class

19

Give your partner a heady experience

Give your partner's head the attention it deserves by lavishing it with extra attention. Start by grasping your partner's shaft firmly with your lubed hand, then try these moves: Hold your mouth over the head and let them feel your warm breath. Swirl your tongue around and over the entire head. Press your tongue into the pee hole. Circle your tongue around the rim and then put your lips around the rim and suck gently. Flick your tongue over the frenulum.

Squeeze a bottle of edible lube and let it drip down slowly, covering their head.

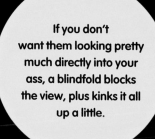

If you don't want them looking pretty much directly into your ass, a blindfold blocks the view, plus kinks it all up a little.

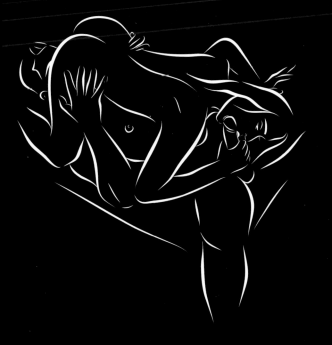

Backwards BJ

20

You look good. Real good.
To give your partner a whole new experience of your mouth and hands, straddle their chest, facing their feet. Lube up your hands and run them down their inner thighs and over their balls, stopping to cup each one gently. Lube their shaft up with your hands. Stroke the lower half of their shaft with your hands while you take the head and top half of their penis in your mouth. Bonus: Excellent view of your ass.

The Tongue Press

21

When they look highly lickable

Press your partner's cock so it's flat up against their belly. Flatten your tongue along the shaft, pressing down with wet firm pressure. Slide your head up and down keeping your tongue pressed and curled around their shaft. Wrap your hand around the base of their shaft as you slide your tongue along their length. As your partner gets closer to coming, squeeze your hand around the base of their cock to mimic the contractions of orgasm.

Use an edible lube for bonus slipperiness that won't taste chemical.

The Two Fister

22

They are so huge you need two hands

You can create the feeling of a vagina or ass—depending on what your partner wants to put their dick into—with just your hands and some lube. Wrap both of your hands around your partner's penis in a prayer position. Make a tunnel with your hand—the lube will help create suction. Use your mouth on their head to extend the feeling of warm wetness. Go ahead and hold on firmly with your hands, it'll make you feel tighter.

A dollop of arousal or stimulation gel for penises can add some extra oomph.

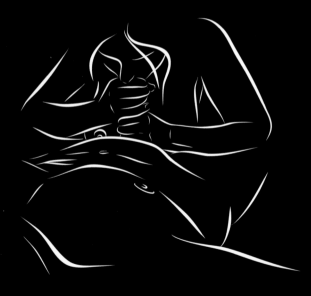

Battery Charged 69

23

Better living through technology

Sometimes the multitasking of a 69 kind of ruins it. How are you supposed to give good oral while simultaneously getting it? Give as good as you get by bringing a toy into it. Lie on your sides facing each other a la traditional 69, but instead of them using their mouth on you, hand them a toy to do the job. They get to focus solely on the feel of your mouth, you get an orgasm. Everyone's happy.

For equal toy opportunity, use a penis stroker on your partner's shaft while you suck on their head.

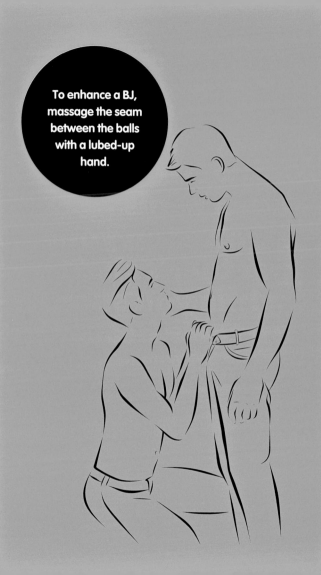

The Ball Handler

24

What to do with that set of balls in front of you

Before you commence the focused suckery that leads to orgasm, give the balls their due. Cup them in your hands and bring your mouth so close they can feel your hot breath. Run your tongue along the line up the middle of the perineum and between the balls (called raphe, if you must know), and up their shaft. Lightly nibble with your lips around the scrotum, then take each ball into your mouth and gently suck.

The Hot Seat

25

Plus an orgasm for you, too

A blow job *and* an orgasm for you?
Yes, please. Have your partner lie
comfortably on their back while you
kneel between their legs to service
them with mouth and tongue. Straddle
a pillow with your favorite vibe propped
on it. (If you're not a vibe person, use
your hand.) As you get more turned on,
you'll translate that passion into a sexier,
more urgent BJ and you get to ride the
wave toward orgasm together. Win win.

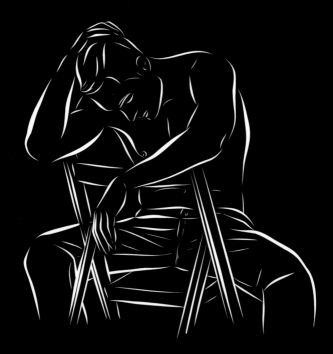

Try a CBD suppository to ease the way and enhance sensations.

P-Gasmic

26

Tap into the power of the prostate

To give your partner next-level pleasure, including stronger, more intense orgasms, get the prostate involved. To unleash its superpowers, suck your partner's penis until they're well aroused. When/if they give you the go-ahead, slide a well-lubed finger into their butt, curling it up against the top wall. Feel for a swollen area, about the size of a walnut about two inches in. As you work on their cock with your mouth, press, rub, and/or tap on the prostate.

Back That Ass Up

27

This sucks ass. No, seriously.
Analingus, a.k.a. a rim job, is basically oral sex for the butt. If y'all are game, a good way for easy access is to have your partner on all fours. Kneel behind them, filling your hand with lube then cupping it over their cock. As you stroke up their shaft and head, kneel down to lick their butt hole. (Yes, analingus is pretty f-ing graphic.) Try circles with a pointed tongue, long licks, and gentle sucks.

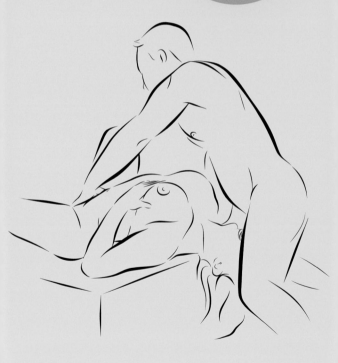

If you're worried about the whole butt aspect of this, try it straight out of the shower.

If you don't want to put your finger in someone else's butt, totally valid. Try putting a condom on your finger.

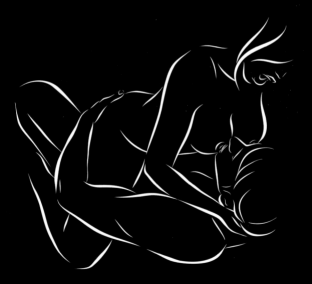

Milking It

28

Got milk?

Prostate milking is massaging the prostate until a milky fluid—it's ejaculate minus the sperm—starts coming out of the penis. Why do this? Amazing orgasm, my friend. Add it to a blow job to enhance the whole experience. As your partner gets closer to orgasm, slide a well-lubed finger into their ass. Press against the upper wall with a steady rhythm. As they orgasm, keep pressing to extend the stellar orgasmic contractions you're giving them.

Supercharged P-Gasm

29

For truly geyser-like orgasms

Trying to suck someone's cock, attend to their balls, *and* give them some P-spot love can be a lot of multitasking. Go ahead and enlist a toy to help out. Start by wrapping your mouth and hands around your partner's cock so they feel fully enveloped by you. As you suck and stroke their cock, fire up a vibrating prostrate toy, cover it in lube, and slide it inside them. Caveat: explosive results. May require protective goggles.

If you don't have
a P-spot toy, put
a G-spot vibrator
on the job.

For a more intense experience, try pressing a rumbly vibe against your partner's perineum just before orgasm.

The Perineum Press

30

Less hardcore P-spot play

If your partner isn't into having anything in their butt, you can still give them the joys of prostate stimulation. Go for it externally by pressing on their perineum, a.k.a. the taint, the area of skin between the balls and the butthole. Stroke and suck their cock until they are clearly into it, then press a lubey finger or thumb onto their perineum as they near and go through orgasm. Keep your finger pressed there or tap firmly, like you're pressing a doorbell.

Quarto.com

© 2024 Quarto Publishing Group
USA Inc.
Text © 2013, 2015, 2024 Jessica O'Reilly

This edition first published in
2024 by Fair Winds Press, an
imprint of The Quarto Group,
100 Cummings Center, Suite 265-D,
Beverly, MA 01915, USA.
T (978) 282-9590 F (978) 283-2742

Fair Winds Press titles are also available
at discount for retail, wholesale,
promotional, and bulk purchase.
For details, contact the Special Sales
Manager by email at specialsales@
quarto.com or by mail at The Quarto
Group, Attn: Special Sales Manager, 100
Cummings Center, Suite 265-D, Beverly,
MA 01915, USA.

28 27 26 25 24   1 2 3 4 5

ISBN: 978-0-7603-9242-3

Digital edition published in 2024
eISBN: 978-0-7603-9243-0

Library of Congress Control Number
available.

Compiled and edited by Jill Hamilton
Design and layout: Burge Agency
Illustration: Sandra Alutyte

Printed in China

The information in this book is for
educational purposes only. Any type of
sexual activity should be consensual.